Healthy Mediterranean Meals Cooking Guide

Super Simple Mediterranean Recipes

Mateo Buscema

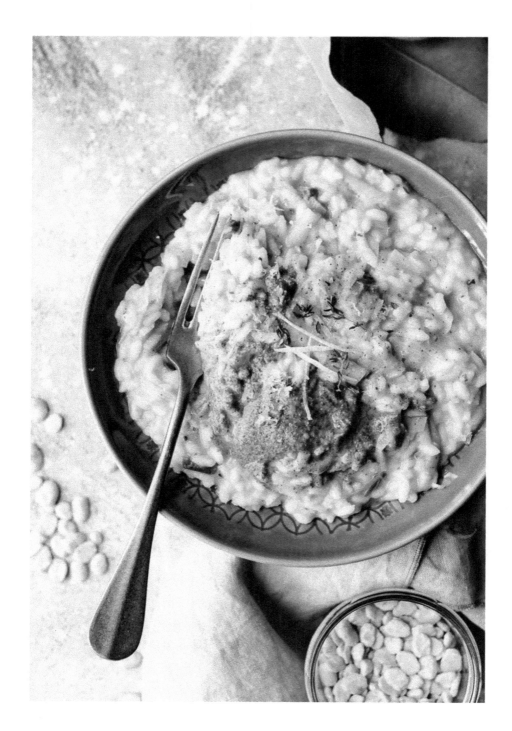

TABLE OF CONTENTS

Easy Mediterranean style shrimp stew

This easy Mediterranean shrimp stew is prepared with chunky yet rustic tomato sauce with wonderful flavor from the garlic, onions, and bell peppers.

Ingredients

- ⅓ cup of toasted pine nuts, optional
- 1 large red onion, chopped
- 1 ½ teaspoon of ground coriander
- 1 bell pepper, cored, chopped
- 5 garlic cloves, chopped
- ¼ cup of toasted sesame seeds
- 1 teaspoon of sumac
- Extra virgin olive oil
- Lemon or lime wedges
- 1 teaspoon of red pepper flakes
- ½ teaspoon of ground green cardamom
- 2 15-oz. cans of diced tomatoes
- ½ cup water
- Kosher salt and black pepper
- 1 teaspoon of cumin

- 2 ½ lb. large shrimp
- 1 cup of parsley leaves

Directions

1. Preheat the oven to 375°F.
2. In a large skillet or frying pan, heat 2 tablespoons of extra virgin olive oil until shimmering but with smoke.
3. Add chopped onions, bell peppers, and garlic.
4. Let cook for 4 minutes, tossing regularly.
5. Stir in spices and continue to cook for 1 more minute.
6. Add diced tomatoes and water.
7. Season with kosher salt and pepper.
8. Boil, then lower heat to let simmer 15 minutes.
9. Transfer sauce to an oven-save dish.
10. Stir shrimp into the sauce.
11. Add parsley together with the pine nuts, and toasted sesame seeds.
12. Tighten the lid with a foil.
13. Transfer to heated oven let bake for 9 minutes.
14. Uncover and broil briefly till shrimp is ready.
15. Serve and enjoy.

Extra creamy avocado hummus recipe

Avocado is the king for skin nourishing among Mediterranean Sea diet recipes. Chickpeas combined with creamy avocado will definitely surprise your taste buds every possible way flavored with garlic, cumin and cayenne.

Ingredients

- ½ lime, juice of lemon
- 2 garlic cloves
- 15-oz. can of chickpeas, drained
- Liquid from canned chickpeas
- ½ teaspoon of cayenne pepper
- 2 tablespoons of Greek Yogurt
- 3 tablespoons of tahini
- Salt
- 2 medium ripe avocados, roughly chopped
- 1 teaspoon of ground cumin

Directions

1. In a large food processor, add the garlic together with the chickpeas, avocados, Greek yogurt, tahini, salt, cumin, cayenne and lime juice.
2. Blend until the hummus mixture is smooth.
3. Taste and adjust everything accordingly.
4. Run the processor again until you achieve the desired creamy consistency. Again adjust seasoning as required.
5. Transfer the avocado hummus to a serving dish and cover tightly with plastic wrap.
6. Chill in a refrigerator before serving.
7. Uncover and smooth the surface of the hummus and drizzle a bit of extra virgin olive oil.
8. Garnish with fresh parsley.
9. Serve and enjoy.

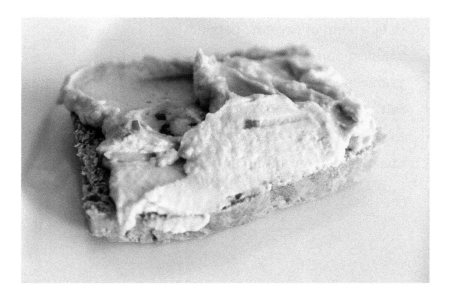

Melitzanosalata recipe

This recipe copes the Greek style of smoky dip of eggplant with aromatics especially garlic, parsley, lemon juice, and extra virgin olive oil.

Ingredients

- ¼ cup of extra virgin olive oil
- 2 large garlic cloves minced
- ¼ red onion finely chopped
- 2 large eggplants
- 1 cup of chopped fresh parsley packed
- Kosher salt and black pepper
- ½ teaspoon of each ground cumin
- A few pitted Kalamata olives sliced
- Feta cheese a sprinkle
- Crushed red pepper flakes
- 1 lemon zested and juiced

Directions

1. Keep the eggplant whole and pierce with a fork in a few places.

2. Place the eggplant over a gas flame or under a broiler, let cook, keep turning using tongs, until the skin is fully charred

3. Cool and drain eggplant.

4. Place the eggplant in a bowl and until cool enough to handle.

5. Peel the charred skins off and discard.

6. Cut into chunks and place in a colander to get rid of any remaining excess juices for 10 minutes.

7. Shift eggplant to a mixing bowl.

8. Add the garlic together with the onion, parsley, lemon juice, olive oil .

9. Add salt and pepper and spices, mix to combine.

10. Break up the eggplant into smaller chunks.

11. Cover the eggplant dip well, let chill in the refrigerator shortly.

12. Transfer the eggplant dip to a serving plate and spread.

13. Drizzle with extra virgin olive oil.

14. Organize and garnish with red onions, lemon zest, parsley, olives, a sprinkle of feta.

15. Serve and enjoy with crusty bread.

Veggie teriyaki stir-fry with noodles

Quick and easy stir fry vegetables with noodles for a healthy dinner is perfect for a Mediterranean Sea diet in 40 minutes max.

Ingredients

- ½ cup teriyaki sauce
- ¼ cup thinly sliced green onion
- 2 tablespoons extra-virgin olive oil
- ½ teaspoon fine sea salt
- 6 cups thinly sliced mixed vegetables*
- 1 to 2 teaspoons toasted sesame oil
- 1 medium red or white onion
- 4 ounces soba noodles, brown rice noodles
- 1 teaspoon sesame seeds

Directions

1. Bring a pot of water to boil.
2. Place the noodles let cook the noodles as per the package Directions.

3. Drain and set aside for later.
4. Warm a large skillet over medium heat.
5. Add the oil, onion, and salt let for 4 – 6 minutes until onions are tender.
6. Add the remaining vegetables and cook until they are tender and caramelizing on the edges in 10 – 15 minutes.
7. Add the noodles and ½ cup of teriyaki sauce to the pan.
8. Stir to combine, let cook till the ingredients are all warmed through in 1 minute.
9. Remove the skillet from the heat source.
10. Add toasted sesame oil together with the sesame seeds.
11. Serve the noodles in bowls with sliced green onion.
12. Sprinkle with sesame seeds on top.
13. Serve and enjoy.

Roasted butternut squash, pomegranate and wild rice stuffing

The recipe can take up to 1 hour and 20 minutes but the sweetness and the health benefit achieved from eating it makes it worth waiting for. It is prepared with kale, wild rice and pomegranate serving from 6 – 12 servings.

Ingredients

- Arils from 1 medium pomegranate,
- 1 tablespoon of maple syrup
- 1 tablespoon of Dijon mustard
- 4 ounces of kale, ribs removed and chopped
- ¾ cup of chopped green onion
- 1 tablespoon of grated fresh ginger
- ½ cup of raw pepitas
- 1 teaspoon of extra-virgin olive oil
- 2 teaspoon of fine sea salt
- 2 tablespoons of apple cider vinegar
- 2 cups of wild rice
- ¼ teaspoon ground cinnamon
- 1 small-to-medium butternut squash

- 2 teaspoon of fine sea salt
- 4 ounces of goat cheese
- ¼ cup of extra-virgin olive oil

Directions

1. Preheat your oven to 425°F.
2. Line a large baking sheet with parchment paper.
3. Bring a large pot of water to boil.
4. Add the rice let cook under reducing heat to simmer for 40 – 55 minutes.
5. Remove from heat, drain, return the rice to the pot
6. Place the cubed butternut squash onto the baking sheet.
7. Drizzle it with the olive oil and a sprinkle of salt.
8. Toss until the cubes are lightly and evenly coated in oil.
9. Arrange them in single layer let roast for 35 – 50 minutes tossing occasionally.
10. Chop the kale and green onion, remove the arils from the pomegranate, whisk together dressing ingredients in a small bowl.
11. combine the pepitas with 1 teaspoon olive oil, ¼ teaspoon of salt and cinnamon in a small skillet stir. Cook for 3 – 5 minutes.
12. Stir in half of the green onions, kale, and ginger dressing.
13. Spread the mixture over a large serving platter.
14. Arrange the butternut squash over the wild rice mixture.

15. Crumble the goat cheese on top with a fork.
16. Top with the toasted pepitas, pomegranate arils, and green onions.
17. Serve while warm and enjoy.

Crispy bean tostadas with smashed avocado and jicama-cilantro slaw

The beans are refried the Mexican way with avocado and cabbage slaw crisp. Prepared with fillings entirely meatless perfect for a Mediterranean Sea diet.

Ingredients

- ½ medium red onion, thinly sliced
- Salt
- Juice of 2 lime
- 6 corn of tortillas
- 2 cups shredded green cabbage
- ½ cup of crumbled queso fresco
- ½ teaspoon ground cumin
- Freshly ground black pepper
- ½ cup fresh cilantro leaves
- Extra-virgin olive oil
- 2 cans of vegetarian refried beans
- 1 tablespoon white vinegar
- ½ teaspoon chili powder
- 3 large ripe avocados, pitted and peeled

- ½ cup ¼-inch-thick slices peeled jicama
- ½ cup of halved grape tomatoes

Directions

1. In a medium bowl, combine the sliced onions together with the lime juice, vinegar and salt stir to coated the onions set aside.
2. In a large bowl, combine the cilantro, cabbage, lime juice, jicama, cumin and chili powder.
3. Season with salt and pepper accordingly.
4. Preheat your oven to 425°F.
5. Brush both sides of the tortilla with olive oil let season with salt.
6. Organize in a single layer on a large baking sheet.
7. Bake for 4 minutes, flip and bake for 4 – 8 minutes, till crispy.
8. Gently heat the refried beans in the microwave.
9. In a large sized bowl, mash the avocados with a fork.
10. Stir in the lime juice and season with salt accordingly.
11. Spread refried beans evenly over every tortilla.
12. Add a layer of smashed avocado and top with the pickled onions, slaw, tomatoes and queso fresco.
13. Serve soon enough and enjoy.

Mango burrito bowls with crispy tofu and peanut sauce

The recipe is prepared with tofu, brown rice, peanut sauce and fresh mango from the tree. It takes max I hour and 15 minutes to get ready.

Ingredients

- ½ cup of sliced green onions
- 1 block of organic extra-firm tofu
- 1 medium red bell pepper, chopped
- 1 tablespoon extra-virgin olive oil
- ¼ cup chopped fresh cilantro
- 3 tablespoon reduced-sodium tamari
- 2 cups shredded cabbage
- ¼ teaspoon fine sea salt
- 1 tablespoon cornstarch
- 1 medium jalapeño, seeds and ribs removed, minced
- 1 ¼ cups brown basmati rice
- ⅓ cup creamy peanut butter
- 5 tablespoons lime juice
- 1 tablespoon honey or maple syrup, to taste
- 2 teaspoons toasted sesame oil

- Handful of chopped roasted peanuts
- 2 garlic cloves, minced
- ¼ teaspoon red pepper flakes
- 2 large ripe mangos

Directions

1. Preheat your oven to 400°F.
2. Align a large baking sheet with parchment paper.
3. Drain the tofu.
4. Slice the tofu into thirds lengthwise in 3 even slabs.
5. Stack the slabs on top of each other and slice through them lengthwise to 3 even columns, slice across to 5 even rows.
6. Arrange the tofu in an even layer on a board with towels.
7. Fold the towel over the cubed tofu.
8. Place something heavy on top to drain.
9. Allow it to rest for at least 10 minutes or accordingly.
10. Bring a large pot of water to boil.
11. Add the rice, boil uncovered for 30 minutes.
12. Drain and return the rice to the pot.
13. Cover the pot let rice simmer for 10 minutes, set aside.
14. Move the pressed tofu to the lined baking sheet.
15. Drizzle with the olive oil and tamari.
16. Toss to combine and sprinkle the starch over the tofu toss again till evenly coated.

17. Arrange the tofu in an even layer.
18. Bake for 25 – 30 minutes toss halfway, until deeply golden on the edges. Set aside.
19. Whisk all the ingredients together in a bowl.
20. Taste and season accordingly, set aside.
21. In a medium mixing bowl, combine the diced mango, bell pepper, green jalapeño, onion, lime juice, cilantro, and salt.
22. Stir to combine, and set aside.
23. Scoop rice top with a handful of shredded cabbage.
24. Add a big scoop of mango salsa, a handful of baked tofu, a hefty drizzle of peanut sauce, and a sprinkle of chopped peanuts.
25. Serve and enjoy

Halloumi tacos with pineapple salsa and aji Verde

Ingredients

- Aji Verde
- 8 small corn
- ¼ cup of extra-virgin olive oil
- Pineapple Salsa
- 8 ounces of halloumi cheese, sliced into rounds

Directions

1. In a medium skillet using a medium heat, warm the tortilla through.
2. Stack them together under a clean tea towel.
3. In the same skillet, warm olive oil over medium heat.
4. Place slices of halloumi into the hot oil.
5. Cook the cheese until golden in 2 – 4 minutes.
6. Flip each piece of cheese with the tongs let cook until the other side is golden 2 – 4 minutes.
7. Place a few paper towels on a cutting board to absorb excess oil.
8. Place cooked cheese onto the plate let cool a bit before handling.

9. Slice each piece of cheese into strips.

10. Place a few strips of cheese along half of your tortilla.

11. Top with pineapple salsa.

12. Finish each taco with a drizzle of aji Verde.

13. Serve warm and enjoy.

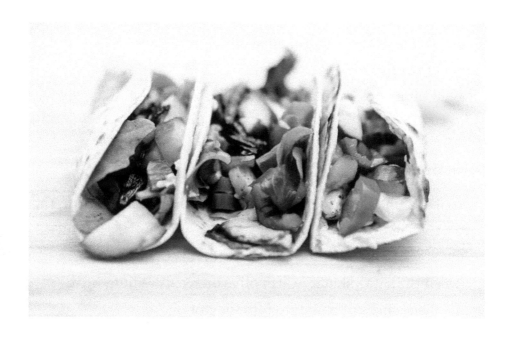

Baked ziti with roasted vegetables

Roasted vegetables are significant in elevating this baked ziti. Prepared with mozzarella, pasta and red sauce, the baked ziti with roasted vegetables is a delicious meal.

Ingredients

- 2 cups of cottage cheese
- 1 red bell pepper
- 8 ounces of ziti, rigatoni
- 2 tablespoons of extra-virgin olive oil
- ¼ teaspoon of fine sea salt
- 1 medium head of cauliflower cut into florets
- 4 cups of marinara sauce
- ¼ cup of chopped fresh basil
- 1 medium yellow onion, wedged
- 8 ounces of grated part-skim mozzarella cheese

Directions

1. Preheat your oven to 425°F.
2. Line two large baking sheets with parchment paper.

3. Place the cauliflower florets on one pan.

4. Combine the bell peppers and onion on the other.

5. Drizzle olive oil over the pans.

6. Sprinkle salt over the two pans.

7. Toss until the vegetables on each pan are lightly coated in oil.

8. Organize the vegetables in an even layer across each pan.

9. Bake for 30 – 35 minutes till the vegetables are tender and caramelized on the edges.

10. Toss the veggies and swapping their rack positions halfway.

11. Bring a large pot of salted water to boil.

12. Cook the pasta according to package instruction.

13. Drain and return to the pot.

14. Add 2 cups of the marinara, the chopped basil, and ½ cup of the mozzarella, stir to combine.

15. Spread 1 cup of marinara sauce inside the baker.

16. Top with half of the pasta mixture, spread into an even layer.

17. Sprinkle the roasted cauliflower on top.

18. Dollop 1 cup of the cottage cheese over the cauliflower and ½ cup of the mozzarella.

19. Top with the remaining pasta.

20. Sprinkle the roasted peppers and onion on top.

21. Dollop the remaining cup of ricotta and marina.

22. Sprinkle the remaining cheese all over.

23. Place the baking sheet on the lower oven rack to catch any drippings.
24. Place the ziti, uncovered, on top of the baking sheet.
25. Bake for 30 minutes
26. Move to the upper rack for 2 – 5 minutes until deeply golden
27. Remove the baker from the oven let cool for 10 minutes.
28. Sprinkle freshly torn basil on top, slice with a knife.
29. Serve and enjoy.

Thai panang curry vegetables

The recipe embraces the health power of vegetable; as such, it is fully packed with vegetables and variety of fresh flavors.

Ingredients

- Fresh Thai basil, sriracha or chili garlic sauce
- 1 tablespoon coconut oil
- 1 to 2 tablespoons panang curry paste
- 1 tablespoon tamari
- Pinch of salt
- ½ cup water
- 1 yellow, orange, sliced into strips
- 3 carrots, peeled and sliced
- 2 cloves garlic, pressed
- 1 can regular coconut milk
- 2 tablespoons peanut butter
- 1 ½ teaspoons coconut sugar
- 1 red bell pepper, sliced into strips
- 1 small white or yellow onion, chopped
- 2 teaspoons fresh lime juice

Directions

1. Bring a large pot of water to boil.
2. Add rice boil for 30 minutes, lower heat and simmer.
3. When ready drain, return the rice to pot.
4. Cover let rest for 10 minutes set aside.
5. Warm a large skillet over medium heat.
6. When hot, add the oil with onion and a sprinkle of salt let cook, stirring often for 5 minutes.
7. Add bell peppers and carrots let cook until bell peppers can be pierced with fork 3 – 5 minutes, stirring occasionally.
8. Add the garlic and curry paste
9. Let cook for 1 minute, while stirring.
10. Add coconut milk together with water, stir to combine.
11. Simmer the mixture over medium heat.
12. Adjust the heat as necessary until the peppers and carrots have softened in 5 – 10 minutes, stirring occasionally.
13. Remove the pot from the heat.
14. Stir in the peanut butter, sugar, tamari, and lime juice.
15. Add salt and season accordingly.
16. Divide rice and curry into bowls and garnish with fresh basil.
17. Serve and enjoy.

Crispy baked tofu

Ingredients

- 1 block of organic extra-firm tofu
- 1 tablespoon of extra-virgin olive oil
- 1 tablespoon of tamari
- 1 tablespoon of cornstarch

Directions

1. Start by preheat your oven to 400°F.
2. Align a large baking sheet with parchment paper.
3. Drain the tofu with you palms to gently squeeze out the water.
4. Slice the tofu into thirds lengthwise.
5. Stack the slabs on top of each other and slice through them lengthwise making 3 even columns.
6. Slice across to make 5 even rows.
7. Get a chopping board with towel.
8. Arrange the tofu in an even layer on the towel cover with a heavy object to drain extra water.
9. Move pressed tofu to a medium mixing bowl
10. Drizzle with the olive oil and tamari.
11. Toss to combine.

12. Sprinkle the starch over the tofu, toss until starch is evenly coated.
13. Bake for 25 – 30 minutes, toss halfway, until deeply golden on edges.
14. Serve and enjoy.

Homemade veggie chili

This recipe features smoky and complex flavors. It emerged from poultry ingredients and vegetable varieties and classic spices to spike its sweetness and delicacy.

Ingredients

- 2 ribs celery, chopped
- ½ teaspoon salt
- 4 cloves garlic, pressed
- Tortilla chips
- 2 tablespoons chili powder
- 1 ½ teaspoons smoked paprika
- 1 teaspoon dried oregano
- 2 tablespoons extra-virgin olive oil
- Sour cream
- 1 large can of diced tomatoes
- 2 cans of black beans, rinsed and drained
- 1 medium red onion, chopped
- 1 large red bell pepper, chopped
- 1 can of pinto beans, rinsed and drained
- Sliced avocado
- 2 cups of vegetable broth
- 1 bay leaf

- 2 medium carrots, chopped
- 2 tablespoons chopped fresh cilantro
- 1 to 2 teaspoons sherry vinegar
- 2 teaspoons ground cumin
- Chopped cilantro

Directions

1. In a large oven warm the olive oil until shimmering without smoke over medium heat.
2. Add the chopped bell pepper, onion, celery, carrot, and ¼ teaspoon of the salt stir to combine.
3. Cook until the vegetables are tender, onion translucent in 7 – 10 minutes, stirring occasionally.
4. Add garlic, cumin, chili powder, smoked paprika and oregano.
5. Cook until fragrant, stirring constantly for 1 minute.
6. Add diced tomatoes, black beans, vegetable broth, pinto beans, and bay leaf.
7. Stir to combine then simmer for 30 minutes.
8. Remove the chili from the heat and discard the bay leaf.
9. Move 1 ½ cups of the chili to a blender, blend till smooth.
10. Pour the mixture back into the pot.
11. Add the chopped cilantro, stir to combine.
12. Stir in the vinegar to taste.
13. Add salt accordingly.
14. Place in bowls serve and enjoy.

Vegetarian stuffed acorn squash

The use of quinoa filling gives this recipe a beautifully tasty flavor that you cannot possibly resist.

Ingredients

- ¼ cup raw pepitas
- ¼ cup chopped green onion
- 1 cup water
- 2 tablespoons extra-virgin olive oil
- ¼ cup chopped parsley
- 1 clove garlic minced
- 2 medium acorn squash
- ½ teaspoon fine sea salt
- 1 tablespoon lemon juice
- ¾ cup grated Parmesan cheese
- ½ cup quinoa, rinsed
- ¼ cup dried cranberries
- ½ cup crumbled goat cheese

Directions

1. Preheat the oven to 400°F.
2. Align a large baking sheet with parchment paper.

3. Slice through the squash up to down, scoop out the seeds and stringy bits inside.
4. Place the squash halves on the parchment pan.
5. Drizzle 1 tablespoon of the olive oil over the squash.
6. Sprinkle with ¼ teaspoon of salt.
7. Rub the oil into the cut sides of the squash, face the cut sides to the pan.
8. Bake until squash is easily pierced through in 30 – 45 minutes.
9. In a separate medium saucepan, combine quinoa with water.
10. Boil over medium-high heat, then lower heat to simmer uncovered for 12 – 18 minutes.
11. Stir in the cranberries when the mixture is off heat.
12. Cover let steam for 5 minutes.
13. In a medium skillet, toast the pepitas over medium heat as you keep stirring frequently, until golden on the edges in 4 – 5 minutes. Keep aside.
14. Put the quinoa mixture into a medium mixing bowl.
15. Add the toasted garlic, pepitas, parsley, onion, lemon juice, the remaining ¼ teaspoon of salt, and 1 tablespoon of olive oil.
16. Stir for even distribution.
17. Taste and season accordingly.
18. Add the Parmesan cheese and goat cheese stir to combine.

19. Turn the cooked squash halves over.

20. Divide the mixture evenly between halves a spoon.

21. Return the squash to the oven let bake for 15 – 18 minutes.

22. Sprinkle the stuffed squash with 1 tablespoon of chopped parsley.

23. Serve warm and enjoy.

Crispy falafel

Ingredients

- ½ teaspoon of ground cumin
- ¼ cup and 1 tablespoon extra-virgin olive oil
- 1 teaspoon of fine sea salt
- ¼ teaspoon of ground cinnamon
- ½ cup of roughly chopped red onion
- ½ cup of packed fresh cilantro
- ½ teaspoon of freshly ground black pepper
- ½ cup of packed fresh parsley
- 1 cup of dried chickpeas

Directions

1. Preheat oven to 375 °F.
2. Pour ¼ cup of the olive oil in a large baking sheet tilt round to evenly coat.
3. Combine chickpeas, onion, garlic, parsley, salt, pepper, cilantro, cumin, cinnamon, and 1 tablespoon of olive oil in a food processor. Blend for 1 minute till smooth.
4. Shape the falafel into small patties, 2 inches wide, ½ inch thick.
5. Place them falafel on the oiled pan.

6. Bake for 25 – 30 minutes ensure to flip over to bake all sides.
7. Serve and enjoy.

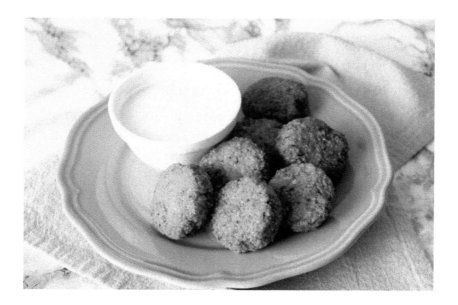

Epic vegetarian tacos

Using pickled onions, refried beans, and avocado sauce, this recipe is so delightfully delicious for a meal with meatless tacos.

Ingredients

- Creamy avocado dip
- 8 corn tortillas
- Quick-pickled onions
- Chopped fresh cilantro
- Lime wedges
- Salsa Verde
- Shredded green cabbage
- Crumbled Cotjia
- Easy refried beans

Directions

1. Prepare these ingredients normally onions, avocado dip, and beans.
2. In a large skillet, warm every side of the tortillas over medium temperature in batches.
3. Stack the warmed tortillas on a plate and cover.
4. Spread refried beans down but at the center of every tortilla.

5. Top with avocado dip and onions.

6. Garnish and serve.

7. Enjoy.

Loaded vegetables nachos

This is a quicker Mediterranean Sea diet veggie with zero percent meat. Prepared with creamy avocado sauce and cheese in 25 minutes.

Ingredients

- 1 packed cup of shredded cheddar cheese
- red bell pepper, chopped
- ⅓ cup crumbled feta cheese
- Your favorite salsa
- 1 can of pinto beans, rinsed and drained
- Avocado dip
- ⅓ cup chopped green onions
- 1 packed cup of shredded Monterey Jack cheese
- 2 radishes, chopped
- Pickled jalapeños
- 2 tablespoons chopped cilantro

Directions

1. Begin by preheating your oven to 400°F.
2. Align a baking sheet with parchment paper.

3. Place handfuls of chips on the baking sheet distributed evenly.
4. Sprinkle the prepared pan of chips evenly with the beans and so the shredded cheese, crumbled feta, bell pepper, and pickled jalapeños.
5. Bake until the cheese is melted in 9 – 13 minutes.
6. When ready, remove, set aside.
7. Drizzle the nachos with avocado sauce.
8. Sprinkle the nachos with radish, onion, and cilantro.
9. Serve soon enough and enjoy when still warm.

Pinto posole

The vegetarian type pinto posole features beans instead of pork.

This recipe is spicy, flavorful and delicious to light up your taste buds.

Ingredients

- ½ teaspoon fine sea salt
- 2 tablespoons extra-virgin olive oil
- 1 lime, halved
- 1 tablespoon ground cumin
- ½ cup of tomato paste
- 1 bay leaf
- 2 cups water
- 3 cans of pinto beans, rinsed and drained
- 2 to 4 guajillo chili peppers
- 1 can of hominy, rinsed and drained
- 32 ounces of vegetable broth
- 4 cloves garlic, pressed or minced
- 1 large white onion, finely chopped
- ¼ cup chopped cilantro

Directions

1. Heat your oven over a medium heat until it evaporates.
2. Toast the chili press flat with a spatula briefly till fragrant flip over repeat.
3. In the same pot, warm the olive oil until shimmering without smoke.
4. Add the onion and a pinch of salt.
5. Cook while stirring frequently, until onions turn translucent in 5 minutes.
6. Add the garlic together with cumin let cook until fragrant in 1 minute.
7. Add the tomato paste cook for 1 minute, keep stirring.
8. Add toasted chili peppers, hominy, bay leaf, vegetable broth, beans, and water to the pot.
9. Stir in salt and raise the heat to medium.
10. Simmer regulate the heat for 25 minutes.
11. Discard the chili peppers and bay leaf..
12. Stir the cilantro and juice of lime into the soup.
13. Taste and season accordingly.
14. Garnish with lime wedges.
15. Serve and enjoy.

Real stovetop mac and cheese

Ingredients

- Tiny pinch of cayenne pepper
- ⅓ cup of heavy cream
- 1 ⅓ packed cups of sharp cheddar cheese
- 8 ounces of regular macaroni noodles
- ⅛ teaspoon of onion powder
- ½ teaspoon of mustard powder
- 2 teaspoons of salt
- ⅛ teaspoon of garlic powder

Directions

1. Bring water to boil in a medium pot.
2. Add noodles and salt.
3. Let cook according to package Directions.
4. Drain the pasta let stay in the colander.
5. Return the same pot heat.
6. Add cream let boil time for 1 minute.
7. Add cheese with spices when the timer is up, stir till cheese has melted.
8. Add boiled pasta, stir to coated in cheese sauce.
9. Remove the pot from the heat source.
10. Taste and season accordingly.

11. Best served and enjoyed immediately.

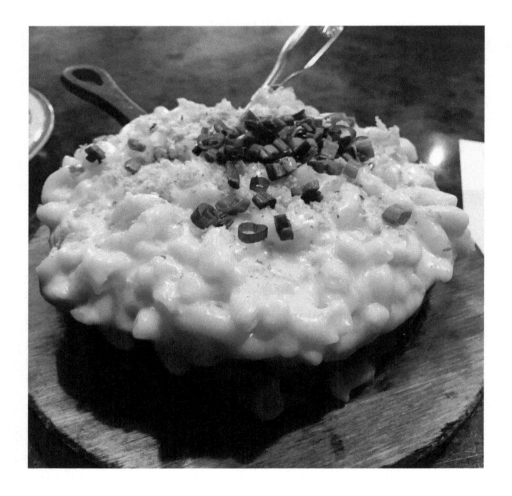

Super simple marinara sauce

With only 5 core ingredients, this marinara sauce is quite simple to make yet very delicious. Here, there is no struggle in chopping this and that because it is not needed.

Ingredients

- Salt
- 1 medium yellow onion
- 2 large cloves garlic left whole
- Pinch of red pepper flakes
- 1 large can of whole peeled tomatoes
- 1 teaspoon of dried oregano
- 2 tablespoons of extra-virgin olive oil

Directions

1. Combine tomatoes, garlic cloves, olive oil, halved onion, oregano and red pepper flakes in a medium saucepan.
2. Simmer over low heat for 45 minutes.
3. Stir occasionally, crush tomatoes with the back of a spoon.
4. Take off the pot from heat source, throw the onion.
5. Stir smashed garlic into the sauce.

6. Add salt season to taste.

7. Serve warm and enjoy.

8. Leftover can be refrigerated for later consumption.

Hearty spaghetti with lentils and marinara

This is a recipe for typical whole meal with lentils, spaghetti, variety of vegetables, and marinara sauce for lunch or dinner. It comes delightfully delicious in only 35 minutes. You can surely wait for that times. Don't you?

Ingredients

- 8 ounces of whole-grain pasta
- 1 bay leaf
- 2 cups of marinara sauce
- 1 large garlic clove, left whole
- ¼ teaspoon of salt
- ½ cup of dry lentils
- 2 cups of vegetable broth

Directions

1. In a small saucepan, combine the bay leaf, garlic, lentils, salt, and broth.
2. Simmer over medium-high heat for 20 – 35 minutes till the lentils have cooked through.

3. Drain the lentils, throw away bay leaf and garlic. Keep uncovered.
4. Boil salted water in a large saucepan.
5. Place in the pasta, cook according to package instruction.
6. Drain, return to the pot keep.
7. Stir the marinara into the lentils, warm over medium heat.
8. Divide pasta into bowls.
9. Top with warm marinara and lentils.
10. Serve and enjoy warm.

Creamy pumpkin marinara

In a period of 25 minutes, this recipe will be read. It readily tastes like fall with comfort just like mac with cheese stuffed with variety of vegetables; of course it is a Mediterranean Sea diet, do not expect anything less vegetarian,

Ingredients

- Finely grated Parmesan and chopped parsley
- 1 red bell pepper, chopped
- ½ teaspoon of dried oregano
- 2 teaspoons of balsamic vinegar
- ¼ teaspoon of dried tarragon
- ¼ teaspoon of ground cinnamon
- 1 can of diced tomatoes
- 1 can of pumpkin purée
- ½ teaspoon of salt, divided
- 2 tablespoons of butter
- 2 cloves garlic, minced
- 2 tablespoons of extra-virgin olive oil
- 1 yellow onion, chopped
- Freshly ground black pepper

Directions

1. In a large skillet, warm olive oil over medium heat.
2. Let shimmer without smoke.
3. Add onion, bell pepper and salt.
4. Let cook while stirring frequently, till onions and pepper are tender in 8 minutes.
5. Add garlic, tarragon, oregano, and cinnamon let cook for 1 minute.
6. Introduce tomatoes let cook for 1 minute.
7. Stir in the pumpkin purée, stir to combine.
8. Simmering for 5 minutes over low heat.
9. Move the mixture to a blender.
10. Add 1 butter together with the vinegar.
11. Blend until very smooth.
12. Season with ground black pepper and salt.
13. Stir in the warm pasta.
14. Serve with grated Parmesan and chopped parsley.
15. Enjoy

Steel cut oat risotto with butternut squash and kale

Ingredients

- 1 ½ cups of Quaker steel-cut oats
- 1 teaspoon salt
- 2 packed cups chopped kale
- ½ cup dry white wine
- Freshly ground black pepper
- 6 cups water
- 1 small butternut squash
- 1 medium red onion, chopped
- ¾ cup of freshly grated Parmesan cheese
- 2 tablespoons butter
- 2 tablespoons extra-virgin olive oil
- 1 tablespoon lemon juice
- Pinch of red pepper flakes
- 4 cloves garlic or minced

Directions

1. Warm olive oil until shimmering without smoke in a medium sized oven.
2. Add butternut, onion, salt, and red pepper flakes.

3. Let cook until the onion is translucent in 8 – 10 minutes.

4. Add garlic together with oats, kale cook to combine in 2 minutes while stirring.

5. Add the wine and scape up with silicone spatula till brown bits form at the bottom.

6. Continue to cook for more 2 minutes keep stirring.

7. Add water and remaining salt.

8. Increased the heat to high let it boil.

9. Lower the heat to allow simmering for 20 – 30 minutes. Ensure the bottom does not scorch

10. Stir in the butter, Parmesan, lemon juice and black pepper.

11. Let rest for 5 minutes.

12. Divide in bowls, serve and enjoy.

Buddha bowl

This is another versatile recipe with rice and variety of fresh vegetables.

Ingredients

- Flaky sea salt
- 1 to 2 tablespoons reduced-sodium tamari or soy sauce
- 4 cups chopped red cabbage
- Sesame seeds
- 2 ripe avocados, halved, pitted sliced into strips
- Toasted sesame oil
- 1 ½ cups frozen shelled edamame
- 1 small cucumber, thinly sliced
- Carrot ginger dressing
- 1 ¼ cups short-grain brown rice
- Thinly sliced green onion
- 1 ½ cups trimmed and roughly chopped snap peas
- Lime wedges

Directions

1. Bring a large pot of water to boil.

2. Add the rice let boil for 25 minutes.

3. Add edamame continue to cook for 3 more minutes.

4. Add snap peas cook for more 2 minutes.

5. Drain excess water when ready.

6. Add veggies and return to the pot.

7. Season with tamari, stir to combine.

8. Divide mixture and raw veggies into 4 bowls.

9. Assemble the cucumber slices along the edge of the bowl.

10. Drizzle lightly with carrot ginger dressing.

11. Top with sliced green onion.

12. Place 2 wedges in each bowl.

13. Divide the avocado into the bowls, then drizzle with sesame oil, sprinkle with sesame seeds and sea salt.

14. Serve and enjoy immediately.

Quick dal makhani

The quick dal makhani is loaded with variety of flavors, and naturally, it is a rich creamy recipe quick to make in 45 minutes.

Ingredients

- 1 medium yellow onion, chopped
- 1 bay leaf
- 1 can of kidney beans
- 1 tablespoon minced fresh ginger
- Chopped fresh cilantro
- 1 jalapeño pepper
- ½ teaspoon of frontier co-op ground cumin
- 2 tablespoons avocado oil
- ½ teaspoon salt
- Freshly ground black pepper
- 1 can of diced tomatoes
- 1 cup of black lentils
- 3 cloves garlic, minced
- ½ teaspoon of frontier co-op ground coriander
- 5 cups of water
- 1 ½ teaspoons of garam masala
- 1 tablespoon lime juice

Directions

1. In a large pot, warm oil until shimmering without smoke over medium heat.
2. Add ginger, onion, garlic, and jalapeño let cook to softened in 4 – 6 minutes. Keep stirring.
3. Stir in the cumin, garam masala, coriander and salt.
4. Season with black pepper.
5. Cook for 1 minute.
6. Add tomatoes cook for 1 minute.
7. Add the lentils together with the kidney beans, water, and bay leaf.
8. Increase the heat to medium-high boil for 20 minutes, lower the heat to simmer for 15 minutes.
9. Move 2 cups of the mixture to a blender.
10. Blend until smooth.
11. Move the mixture to the pot, stir to combine.
12. Add lime juice and season to taste with salt and pepper.
13. Serve in bowls, with chopped cilantro and a lime wedge on top.
14. Serve with rice and enjoy.

Vegetable paella

This vegetable is loaded with smoky rice and savory making it perfect for dinner parties. It is gluten free; thus vegetarian and fit for a Mediterranean Sea diet.

Ingredients

- 1 ½ teaspoons fine sea salt
- 2 tablespoons of lemon juice
- 2 red bell peppers, stemmed, seeded and sliced
- 6 garlic cloves, minced.
- 1 can of diced tomatoes
- ½ cup of frozen peas
- 2 cups of brown rice
- 1 can of chickpeas
- ¼ cup of chopped fresh parsley
- 3 cups of vegetable broth
- ⅓ cup dry white wine
- ½ teaspoon saffron threads
- 1 can of quartered artichokes
- 2 teaspoons smoked paprika
- ½ cup of Kalamata olives
- 1 medium yellow onion.
- 3 tablespoons extra-virgin olive oil

- Freshly ground black pepper.

Directions

1. Preheat your oven to 350°F.
2. Heat 2 tablespoons of oil in your over medium heat to shimmer without smoke.
3. Add onion and a pinch of salt.
4. Let cook until the onions are tender in 5 minutes.
5. Carefully, stir in garlic and paprika let cook until fragrant in 30 seconds.
6. Stir in tomatoes let cook until the mixture darkens somehow in 2 minutes.
7. Stir in the rice and cook until the grains are well coated in 1 minute.
8. Add the chickpeas, wine, broth, saffron, and 1 teaspoon salt.
9. Increase the heat to medium let boil, stirring occasionally.
10. Cover the pot, transfer to lower rack, let bake, till liquid is fully absorbed in 30 − 35 minutes.
11. Align a large baking sheet with parchment paper.
12. Combine the artichoke, chopped olives, peppers, bit of olive oil, salt, and ground black pepper, toss briefly.
13. Spread the mixture across the pan.

14. Roast the vegetables on the upper rack contents are tender in 40 - 45 minutes.
15. Remove from oven, add parsley with lemon juice, toss.
16. Season with salt and pepper. Keep.
17. Sprinkle peas and roasted vegetables over baked rice.
18. Cover to settle paella for 5 minutes.
19. Serve and enjoy.

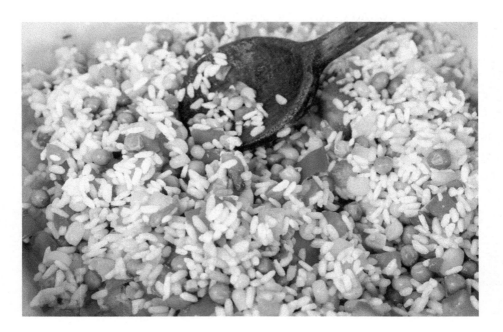

One pan baked cod and vegetables

Ingredients

- 3 - 4 tablespoon of oil of choice
- 1 pound of Atlantic cod divided into 4 pieces
- 2 cups of purple potatoes diced
- 2 cups of Cherry Tomatoes

Directions

1. Begin by preheating your oven to 400°F.
2. Toss diced potatoes with in oil
3. Roast for 15 minutes in the preheated oven.
4. Remove pan from the oven to add in tomatoes and cod.
5. Drizzle with remaining oil and season accordingly.
6. Take back to the oven let it bake for more 10 – 12 minutes
7. Serve and enjoy.

Quinoa bowls with roasted pepper

This recipe blends variety of veggies and herbs with quinoa, cheese, pepperoncini and olives for a delicious meal that you will not forget in ages.

Ingredients

- 1 clove garlic
- Hummus
- ½ teaspoon salt
- Sliced red onion
- ½ cup olive oil
- Pepper
- Kalamata olives
- Cooked quinoa
- Spinach, kale, or cucumber
- Juice of one lemon
- Feta cheese
- Pepperoncini
- ½ cup almonds
- Fresh basil or parsley
- 1 16 ounce of jar roasted red peppers, drained

Directions

1. Combine red pepper, garlic, salt, lemon juice, olive oil, and almonds in a food processor.
2. Blend until smooth.
3. Next cook the quinoa according to package Directions.
4. Build a Mediterranean Quinoa Bowl.
5. Serve and enjoy.

Sweet potato wedges with tahini

This fried potato wedges make a perfect healthy snack. You can choose to dip in a sauce of your choice. The spices used here are almost addictive keeping you hooked onto eating every time and every time.

Ingredients

- ½ teaspoon of smoked paprika
- ½ teaspoon of olive oil
- 2 medium sweet potatoes
- ½ teaspoon of Chili Powder
- Salt and pepper
- ½ teaspoon of cumin
- 2 teaspoon of runny tahini

Directions

1. Preheat your oven to 400°F.
2. Align a baking sheet with parchment paper inside.
3. Cut sweet potatoes in half, then each into 4 – 6 wedges.
4. Organize the wedges on the baking sheet.
5. Drizzle with the olive oil.

6. Then sprinkle with salt, chili powder, pepper, and smoke paprika.
7. Roast in the oven until brown and crispy in 35 – 40 minutes.
8. Remove from the oven, let cool briefly.
9. Serve and enjoy with runny tahini.

Armenia losh kebab

Unlike the common kebabs one can find in any restaurant around the corner, the Armenia losh kebabs are rare to find. You be lucky to find one in a restaurant menu. So use this recipe to make for yourself this delicious kebab.

Ingredients

- 1 cup of fresh parsley, chopped
- 1 lb. of ground beef
- ¾ cup of chopped parsley
- ½ white onion, chopped
- 1 lb. of ground lamb
- 1 white onion, chopped
- 1 tablespoon of cumin
- Juice of ¼ lemon
- 1 tablespoon of extra virgin olive oil
- 1 egg
- ¼ cup of tomato sauce
- Salt and pepper

Directions

1. In a bowl, combine ground beef together with the lamb, onion, egg, parsley, lemon, cumin, olive oil, tomato sauce, salt and pepper.
2. Form into burger patties keep for later.
3. Next, heat your grill to medium high heat.
4. Grill the burgers, make sure to flip once. Put aside to rest.
5. Chop the remaining onion and parsley place in a bowl and let combine.
6. Put your burger in a pita wrap.
7. Use the parsley and onion mixture for topping. Wrap.
8. Enjoy.

Eggplant, lentils and pepper cooked in olive oil

This is another 100 percent vegetarian recipe for a perfect Mediterranean Sea diet packed with bright flavors to tease your taste buds.

Ingredients

- 2 medium eggplants
- 1 red bell pepper, cut in half and thinly sliced
- Freshly ground black pepper
- 2 medium onions, halved and thinly sliced
- 14 ounces can of diced tomatoes
- 7 tablespoons of extra virgin olive oil
- 6 ounces of green lentils, rinsed
- 1 cup of water
- 1 teaspoon of salt
- 2 teaspoons of dried mint
- 4 cloves of garlic, crushed and finely chopped
- 1 teaspoon of granulated sugar

Directions

1. Place in a boiling water to simmer when covered for 15 minutes.
2. Drain out any excess water. Keep aside for later.
3. Peel the eggplant and cut in half lengthwise.
4. Spread on a wide tray then sprinkle with salt keep for 15 minutes.
5. Drain excess water in the eggplants using a pepper towel.
6. Next, heat olive oil 3 teaspoons in a pan, Sauté briefly for 2 minutes.
7. In a large bowl, combine half way cooked lentils with the onion, bell peppers, garlic, tomatoes, dried mint, salt, olive oil, and sugar.
8. Season with black pepper to taste.
9. In another pan, place a layer of eggplant slices.
10. Spread evenly with half of the vegetable mixture.
11. Top with the remaining.
12. Add water let cook for 36 minutes while covered over low heat.
13. Serve and enjoy with crusty breads.

Potato omelet

Ingredients

- 10 eggs
- 1 onion, sliced in rounds, same thickness as potatoes
- ¾ cup extra virgin olive oil
- Salt and pepper
- 4 potatoes, peeled and sliced into rounds

Directions

1. Add olive oil in a skillet frying pan.
2. Add sliced potatoes when the oil is hot enough.
3. Turn occasionally until it changes color to brown.
4. Add onions to the potatoes after 10 minutes of frying.
5. Sprinkle with salt and pepper.
6. Fry further until tender all way through.
7. In another large separate bowl, add the eggs, whisk until smooth.
8. Turn on broiler in oven.
9. Transfer content to a bowl.
10. Let cool.
11. Add oil in the skillet to covered every part in the skillet.
12. Add potato mixture to egg mixture in bowl blend.
13. Add salt and ground black pepper to the mixture.

14. Place in the skillet.

15. Cook until eggs start to set on bottom over medium heat.

16. Continue to cook in the top rack of oven till eggs are set

17. Remove, serve and enjoy.

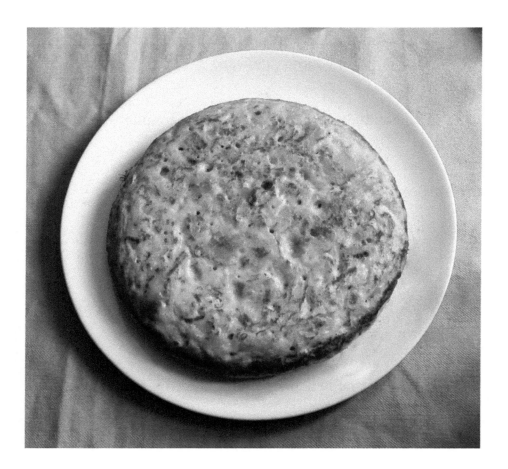

Eggs poached in spicy tomato sauce, the Moroccan style

Ingredients

- 1 teaspoon of cumin
- 2 tablespoons of extra virgin olive oil
- Salt and pepper
- 3 cloves garlic, chopped
- 4 – 6 eggs
- 4 tomatoes of chopped
- 1 red pepper, chopped
- 1 onion, chopped
- ¼ cup fresh oregano, chopped
- 1 jalapeno of pepper, chopped
- 1 teaspoon of smoked paprika

Directions

1. Heat oil in a medium skillet.
2. Sauté onion together with the garlic for 1 minute.
3. Next, add the red pepper. Sauté for 2 minutes.
4. Add jalapeno pepper and also sauté for 30 seconds max.
5. Add cumin, tomatoes, and smoked paprika to simmer for 15 – 20 minutes.

6. Season with salt and pepper.

7. Gently stir in oregano.

8. Finally, break the eggs pour to mixture.

9. Continue to simmer until the egg begins to set.

10. Add more salt and pepper, to taste.

11. Serve and enjoy.

Briam baked vegetables in olive oil

Ingredients

- 1 cup feta, crumbled
- 3-4 small zucchini, ends cut off and cut into pieces
- 2 onions, cut in half
- 1 teaspoon salt
- 1 red pepper, cut into pieces
- 1 orange pepper, cut into large pieces
- 4 small or 2 large potatoes, peeled cut into pieces
- 2 tomatoes, chopped
- 1 bunch dill, chopped
- 2 small or 1 large eggplant, cut into large strips
- ½ cup extra virgin olive oil

Directions

1. Preheat oven to 400°F.
2. In a large baking dish, mix all ingredients apart from feta.
3. Cover with a lid, let bake for 1 hour as your keep stirring occasionally.
4. Stir in feta cheese when off the heat.
5. Serve immediately.
6. And enjoy.

Eggplant parmesan with prosciutto

It is a lot of fun to prepare this recipe traditional style with no bread crumbs with lettuce, tomatoes, and cucumber for a healthy Mediterranean meal in about 1 hour.

Ingredients

- 2 medium sized eggplants
- Olive oil
- Salt and pepper
- Butter
- 1 Cup of tomato sauce
- 6 ounces of thinly sliced, raw Parma Ham
- 1 Cup of grated Parmesan cheese

Directions

1. Begin by simmering the tomato sauce over low heat.
2. Whereas, prepare the eggplant, cut into rounds.
3. Sprinkle with salt, put in a colander for 20 minutes, wash, at dry.

4. Heat olive oil in a saucepan and place the eggplant slices to fry on every slide until brown.
5. Using a paper towel, dry off.
6. Place a layer of eggplant slices at the bottom of a buttered baking bowl.
7. Cover with ham, pepper, tomato sauce, and Parmesan cheese.
8. Repeat until ingredients are used up.
9. Bake in a slow oven at 325°F after dotting with butter on the surface for 1 hour.
10. Serve and enjoy when still hot.

Lebanese hummus

This is another traditional recipe of the Mediterranean Sea diet prepared with garlic, extra virgin olive oil, lemon juice and paprika for a tasty meal to remember.

Ingredients

- 2 garlic cloves, crushed
- pine nuts for garnish
- 3 tablespoon of cold water
- 1/3 cup of freshly squeezed lemon juice
- ¼ cup of extra virgin olive oil
- ¼ teaspoon of paprika
- 2 -15 oz. cans of chickpeas, drained and rinsed
- ¼ cup of tahini paste
- ½ teaspoon of salt

Directions

1. Begin by chopping the garlic and place in a food processor.
2. Add the rest of the remaining ingredients.
3. Blend until desired consistency.
4. Serve and enjoy when smooth.

Grilled swordfish with lemon parsley topping

The lemon used in preparing this dish gives it all the flavor you are seeking for. It is quite easy to make in 10 minutes.

Ingredients

- Salt and pepper
- ½ cup of chopped parsley
- ½ cup of chopped onions
- ½ cup of extra virgin olive oil
- 1 ½ pounds of swordfish steaks
- ½ cup of fresh lemon juice

Directions

1. Wash and pat dry the swordfish.
2. combine onions, olive oil, lemon juice, parsley, salt and pepper in a small bowl.
3. Place on the until firm to the touch in 5 minutes.
4. Remove, then top with lemon parsley mixture.
5. Serve and enjoy.

Orange lemon potatoes

This lemon potatoes recipe uses garlic, oregano, thyme, and lemon juice among others for a flavorful meal.

Ingredients

- Salt and pepper, to taste
- ½ cup of freshly squeezed lemon juice
- 1 cup of water
- 1 clove garlic, minced
- 2 tablespoons of mustard
- 1 ½ pounds of potatoes, peeled cut to quarters
- ½ teaspoon of dried oregano
- 1 cup of freshly squeezed orange juice
- ¾ cup of extra virgin olive oil
- ½ teaspoon of dried thyme

Directions

1. Preheat your oven to 350°F.
2. Add every ingredient to a baking pan.
3. Mix with hands.
4. Salt and pepper accordingly.
5. Bake until potatoes are golden brown.
6. Serve and enjoy.

Chickpea patties with sesame, cilantro and parsley

Ingredients

- 1 leek, cut into small chunks
- Extra virgin olive oil
- 1 bunch parsley, stems removed
- 1 onion cut into quarters
- 1 tablespoon dry coriander powder
- 1 pound dried chickpeas, soaked overnight
- 6 cloves garlic
- ½ teaspoon cumin
- 1 bunch cilantro, stems removed
- Salt and pepper
- 1 tablespoon baking soda
- Sesame seeds

Directions

1. Rinse and drain soaked chickpeas.
2. Add garlic, parsley, leek, onion, and cilantro to a food processor.
3. Process until onion and garlic are pulverized.

4. To the food processor, add the chickpeas with baking soda, coriander powder, cumin, salt and pepper.
5. Ensure not to over blend the mixture.
6. Place mixture in a refrigerator for not less than an hour.
7. Form flat patties out of the mixture.
8. Roll in sesame seeds.
9. Add extra virgin olive oil to a frying pan, let heat over medium temperature.
10. Fry patties until brown on every side.
11. Drain on paper towels.
12. Serve immediately and enjoy.

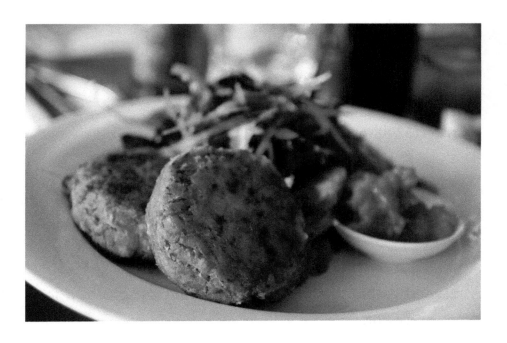

Shrimp with feta and tomatoes

Ingredients

- Salt and pepper, to taste
- 1 red pepper, thinly sliced
- ½ pound of feta, cut into small cubes
- 1 large onion, sliced
- ¼ cup extra virgin olive oil
- 2 cloves garlic, minced
- 2 fresh tomatoes, cut into small cubes
- 1 pound of medium sized shrimp, shells removed and de-veined

Directions

1. In a large heavy frying pan, sauté the onion together with the pepper, and garlic for 5 minutes in olive oil.
2. Add the tomatoes let it simmer for 15 minutes.
3. Add the shrimp and cook for 10 minutes over medium heat.
4. Add the feta also let it simmer for 5 minutes or so.
5. Salt and pepper.
6. Serve and enjoy.

Seared scallops with lemon orzo

It is worth serving this impressive meal with green salad, garlic and white wine. The scallops are seared with orzo for a tastier meal.

Ingredients

- Cooking spray
- 1 ½ pounds of sea scallops
- ¼ teaspoon of black pepper
- 1 cup of uncooked orzo
- 2 teaspoons of olive oil
- 1 cup of fat-free, less-sodium chicken broth
- ½ cup of dry white wine
- ¼ teaspoon of salt
- ¼ teaspoon of dried thyme
- 2 tablespoons of fresh lemon juice
- ½ cup of chopped onion
- 2 tablespoons of chopped fresh chives

Directions

1. Start by heating a medium saucepan over medium temperature coated with cooking spray.

2. Add onion to pan and sauté for 3 minutes.
3. Place in the pasta, wine, broth, and thyme let boil at reduced heat to simmer for 15 minutes to absorb all the liquid.
4. Place in the chopped chives with the lemon juice.
5. Heat oil in another large skillet over medium heat.
6. Sprinkle scallops evenly with salt and pepper.
7. Then add them to the pan let cook for 3 minutes until done.
8. Serve and enjoy with the pasta mixture.

Pasta with sundried tomato pesto and feta cheese

This is a simplified pasta dish with vegetables especially dry tomatoes, almond, garlic and herbs mainly basil. It makes a perfect spiced meal with rich flavor consistence.

Ingredients

- ½ teaspoon of salt
- ¾ cup of oil-packed sun-dried tomato halves, drained
- ½ cup of crumbled feta cheese
- 2 tablespoons of shredded Parmesan cheese
- 1 tablespoon of bottled minced garlic
- ¼ cup of packed basil leaves
- 2 tablespoons of slivered almonds
- ¼ teaspoon of black pepper

Directions

1. Begin by cooking pasta as per the package directions
2. Drain any excess water. Remember to keep 1 cup of the cooking liquid.
3. Return pasta to the cooking pan.

4. Put tomatoes together with basil leaves, almond, parmesan cheese, garlic, and salt in a food processor as the pasta cooks.
5. Process until all chopped.
6. Combine tomato mixture with the pasta water.
7. Stir and whisk.
8. Then, add to pasta and toss.
9. Sprinkle feta on top.
10. Serve and enjoy.

Linguine with garlicky clams and peas

The linguine with garlicky clams and peas recipe is tossed with vegan green salad to spice the whole meal. It draws its flavorful aroma from the garlic and basil among other flavors.

Ingredients

- 2 tablespoons of chopped fresh basil
- 2 tablespoons of olive oil
- 3 cans of chopped clams, undrained
- ¼ cup of dry white wine
- 1 ½ teaspoons of bottled minced garlic
- ¼ teaspoon of crushed red pepper
- 1 package of fresh linguine
- 1 cup of frozen green peas
- 1 cup of organic vegetable broth
- ½ cup of shredded Parmesan cheese

Directions

1. Cook pasta as per the package directions.
2. Drain any excess water.

3. Secondly, heat oil in a large skillet over medium-high heat.
4. Add to garlic to sauté for 1 minute.
5. Drain clams but keep at least 1 cup of the cooking water for later.
6. Add reserved water to broth, wine, and pepper in the pan and boil.
7. Lower heat to simmer for 5 minutes as you stir infrequently.
8. Add clams with peas let cook for 2 minutes.
9. Add pasta and toss.
10. Sprinkle with cheese and basil.
11. Serve and enjoy.

Toum garlic sauce

It is a smooth garlic sauce with garlic flavor throughout the sauce. It is versatile enough to spread and eat with anything whether shawarma, kofta, and falafel among others.

Ingredients

- 1 ¾ cups of grape seed oil or sunflower oil
- 1 teaspoon of kosher salt
- 6 tablespoon of ice water
- 1 head garlic
- 1 lemon juice

Directions

1. Peel the garlic cloves. Cut the cloves in half and remove the green germ.
2. Place the garlic and kosher salt in the bowl of a food processor.
3. Pulse a briefly until the garlic looks minced, scrape down the sides as you process.
4. Add the lemon juice and pulse a few times to combine.
5. Drizzle with oil in as the processor is still running.
6. Add in 1 tablespoon of the ice water.

7. Stop to scrape down the sides of the processor bowl.

8. Keep the processor running as you continue to slowly drizzle in the oil.

9. Endeavor to add a tablespoon of the ice water after every ¼ cup of oil.

10. Continue with this process until you have used up all the oil.

11. Serve and enjoy.

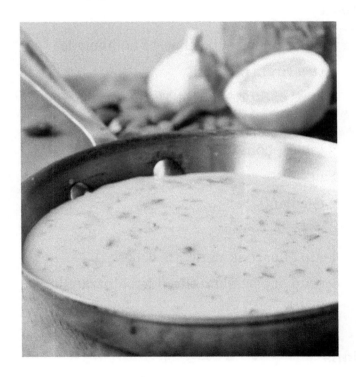

Eggplant rollatini recipe

This recipe uses a tasty part-skim ricotta cheese filling with herbs parked in red sauce to tease you taste buds. It is a perfect Mediterranean Sea vegetarian diet.

Ingredients

- 2 tablespoons of basil pesto homemade
- Extra virgin olive oil
- 2 cups of Store-bought Marinara sauce
- 1 cup chopped fresh parsley leaves
- 3 tablespoons of grated Parmesan
- Salt
- 2 eggplants
- 2 eggs beaten
- 1 cup of part-skim ricotta cheese
- ½ cup of part-skim shredded Mozzarella

Directions

1. Start by slicing the eggplants length-wise.
2. Sprinkle eggplant slices with salt and keep aside on paper towel for 20 minutes.
3. Pat dry. Rinse with water, then dry again.

4. Heat your oven to 375°F.

5. Brush a large baking sheet with extra virgin olive oil.

6. Organize the eggplant slices in one layer on baking sheet.

7. Brush the tops of the eggplant slices with more extra virgin olive oil.

8. Bake in heated oven for 8 minutes until soft enough to fold.

9. Remove from oven let cool shortly.

10. In a bowl, add eggs together with the ricotta, grated Parmesan, Mozzarella, basil pesto, and fresh parsley. Mix to combined.

11. Spread ¾ cup marinara sauce on the bottom of a baking dish.

12. Scoop 2 tablespoons of the filling onto one end of each eggplant slice.

13. Spread, starting from the short end, roll up eggplant slices tightly and arranged on prepared baking dish.

14. Top eggplant rollatini with the remainder of the marinara sauce and a sprinkle of mozzarella.

15. Bake in heated oven for 30 minutes until tender.

16. Remove from oven let settle for 10 minutes.

17. Serve and enjoy.

Vegetarian moussaka recipe

This recipe is also eggplant based entailing layers of roasted eggplants, zucchini, and potatoes with delicious Mediterranean tomato lentil soup.

Ingredients

- Salt
- 2 large zucchinis, sliced length-wise
- Extra virgin olive oil
- ½ teaspoon of nutmeg
- ⅔ cup of all-purpose flour
- Pinch of cinnamon
- 1 teaspoon of dry oregano
- 2 medium eggplants partially peeled and sliced length-wise
- ½ teaspoon of salt, more if you like
- ¼ teaspoon of ground nutmeg
- 4 cups of milk, warmed
- 2 large eggs
- 1 yellow onion, chopped
- 3 Russet potatoes, peeled and sliced lengthwise
- 2 garlic cloves, minced
- 1 ¼ cup of cooked black lentils

- 1 14-oz. can of crushed tomatoes
- ⅓ cup + 2 tablespoons of Greek extra virgin olive oil
- ½ cup of broth or water

Directions

1. Heat your oven to 400°F.
2. Spread eggplant slices on a large pan lined with paper towel and sprinkle with kosher salt, set aside for 20 to 30 minutes.
3. Pat dry with paper towels
4. In a large saucepan, heat olive oil over medium-high heat until shimmering without smoke.
5. Stir in flour together with the salt and pepper let cook until golden.
6. Gradually add the warmed milk, whisking continuously.
7. Continue cooking, stirring occasionally, over medium heat for 7 minutes.
8. Add nutmeg and in a small bowl, whisk a small amount of the hot béchamel mixture with the 2 eggs.
9. Then return all to the pan with the balance of the béchamel mixture.
10. Continue to whisk, then boil for 2 minutes.
11. Taste and adjust salt and pepper.
12. Remove from heat let allow to cool.

13. In a large non-stick pan, heat 1 tablespoon of extra virgin olive oil over medium heat.
14. Sauté onions together with the garlic briefly, tossing regularly.
15. Stir in cooked black lentils together with the crushed tomatoes and broth.
16. Season with a dash of kosher salt.
17. Add oregano, nutmeg and a small pinch of ground cinnamon.
18. Boil, then lower heat and cover part-way let simmer for 20 minutes.
19. While lentil sauce is simmering, bake the vegetables. Arrange the potatoes, zucchini and eggplant slices on lightly oiled baking sheets. Brush with extra virgin olive oil. Bake in heated oven for 15 to 20 minutes just until tender.
20. Pour bit of the lentil sauce on the bottom of the baking dish and spread.
21. Layer the vegetables on top.
22. Add the remainder of the lentil sauce and spread béchamel sauce on top, ensure it is smooth.
23. Place moussaka casserole on the middle rack of your heated oven let bake for 45 minutes.
24. Remove from heat, let sit for at 30 minutes before cutting.
25. Serve and enjoy.

Honey mustard salmon recipe

This salmon is quite flaky covered or coated with sweet natural honey mustard sauce. It is flavored with garlic featuring other vegetables mainly paprika and cayenne.

Ingredients

- 2 ½ teaspoon of Extra virgin olive oil
- Lime wedges to serve
- ½ teaspoon of black pepper
- ½ teaspoon of cayenne
- Parsley garnish
- 4 tablespoons of whole grain mustard
- 2 tablespoons of honey
- 2 lb.. salmon fillet
- Kosher salt
- 4 garlic cloves minced
- 1 teaspoon of smoked paprika

Directions

1. Firstly, heat your oven to 375°F.
2. Pat dry the salmon fillet.
3. Season with salt on both sides.

4. In a small bowl, whisk together honey with whole grain mustard, minced garlic, extra virgin olive oil, smoked paprika, cayenne, and black pepper.
5. Place the salmon on a lightly oiled sheet pan.
6. Spread the honey mustard sauce evenly over the surface of the salmon.
7. Cover with an aluminum foil bake for 20 minutes.
8. Place under the broiler for 3 minutes uncovered.
9. Place the seasoned salmon on a large, lightly oiled piece of aluminum foil.
10. Spread the honey mustard sauce on top of the salmon.
11. Fold both sides of the foil over the salmon and tightly close at the top.
12. Place on a medium-high gas grill.
13. Let cook for 10 – 12 minutes when covered.
14. Open the top of the foil up so the fish is exposed.
15. Cook for 3 more minutes.
16. Remove from the heat source and squeeze a bit of fresh lime juice and garnish with parsley.
17. Serve and enjoy.

Muhammara recipe/roasted red pepper dip

This is perfect substation or addition to the mezze table with baba ganoush and hummus served with pita bread or chips.

Ingredients

- 1 teaspoon of Aleppo pepper
- ¼ lb. shelled toasted walnuts
- ½ teaspoon of cayenne pepper
- ½ teaspoon of salt
- 1 garlic clove roughly chopped
- 2 ½ tablespoons of tomato paste
- ¾ cup of bread crumbs
- 2 tablespoons of molasses
- ½ teaspoon of sugar
- 4 tablespoons of extra virgin olive oil divided
- 2 red bell peppers
- 1 teaspoon of sumac

Directions

1. Preheat your oven to 425°F.

2. Brush the bell peppers with bit of olive oil.

3. Place in a lightly oiled oven pan.

4. Roast for 30 minutes turn over occasionally.

5. Remove and place the peppers in a bowl.

6. Cover with plastic wrap for a few minutes.

7. When cool enough to handle, peel the peppers, remove the seeds and slice the peppers into small strips.

8. In the bowl of a large food processor, combine the roasted red pepper strips together with 3 tablespoons of extra virgin olive oil, tomato paste, walnuts, bread crumbs, Aleppo pepper, pomegranate molasses, sugar, sumac, salt and cayenne.

9. Blend into a smooth paste.

10. Transfer to a serving bowl.

11. Serve and top with a drizzle of extra virgin olive oil, and garnish with walnuts and fresh parsley, if desired.

12. Enjoy with pita chips.

Mediterranean grain bowl recipe with lentils and chickpeas

Ingredients

- 2 ½ tablespoons of fresh lemon juice
- Salt
- 1 zucchini squash, sliced into rounds
- 3 cups cooked faro
- 2 cups of cooked brown lentils
- 2 cups of cooked chickpeas
- ½ teaspoons of ground Sumac
- 2 ½ teaspoons of quality Dijon mustard
- 1 teaspoon of Za'atar spice
- Extra virgin olive oil
- 2 cups of cherry tomatoes, halved
- 2 shallots, sliced
- 1 cup of fresh chopped parsley
- Handful pitted Kalamata olives
- Sprinkle of crumbled feta cheese
- 2 avocados, skin removed, pitted and sliced
- 1 garlic clove, minced
- Salt and pepper

Directions

1. In a skillet, heat 2 tablespoons of olive oil over medium heat until shimmering but without smoke.

2. Add the sliced zucchini and sauté on both sides until tender.

3. Remove zucchini and place on a paper towel to drain any excess oil.

4. Season with salt.

5. Add the extra virgin olive oil, lemon juice, garlic, salt and pepper, za'atar spice, and sumac to a mason jar.

6. Close tightly, and give it a good shake. Set aside for later.

7. Divide the cooked faro, lentils, and chickpeas equally among four dinner bowls.

8. Add cooked zucchini, tomatoes, shallots, avocado slices, parsley, and Kalamata olives.

9. Season with salt, pepper and za'atar then drizzle a bit of the dressing on top.

10. Serve and enjoy at room temperature.

Roasted cauliflower and chickpea stew

This is a perfect match for serving over couscous or rice. The cauliflower is deliciously roasted and loaded with carrots, cumin, tomatoes, cinnamon and paprika for a Mediterranean dish.

Ingredients

- ½ cup of parsley leaves, stems removed, roughly chopped
- 1 ½ teaspoons of ground turmeric
- 1 28-oz. can of diced tomatoes with its juice
- 1 ½ teaspoons of ground cumin
- 1 ½ teaspoons of ground cinnamon
- 1 teaspoon of Sweet paprika
- Toasted pine nuts
- 2 14-oz. cans of chickpeas, drained and rinsed
- 1 teaspoon of cayenne pepper
- ½ teaspoon of ground green cardamom
- 1 whole head cauliflower, divided into small florets
- 5 medium-sized bulk carrots, peeled, cut pieces
- Salt and pepper
- Extra virgin olive oil

- Toasted slivered almonds
- 1 large sweet onion, chopped
- 1 teaspoon of ground coriander
- 6 garlic cloves, chopped

Directions

1. Preheat the oven to 475°F.
2. In a small bowl, mix together the spices.
3. Place the cauliflower florets and carrot pieces on a large lightly oiled baking sheet.
4. Season with salt and pepper.
5. Add some spice mixture.
6. Drizzle with olive oil, then toss to coat.
7. Bake for 20 minutes in the preheated oven or until the carrots and cauliflower soften.
8. Remove from the heat and keep for later. Turn the oven off.
9. In a large cast iron pot , heat 2 tablespoons of olive oil.
10. Add the onions and sauté for 3 minutes, add the garlic and the remaining spices.
11. Let cook for 3 minutes on medium-high heat, stirring constantly.
12. Add chickpeas with the canned tomatoes.
13. Season with salt and pepper.
14. Stir in the roasted cauliflower and carrots boil.

15. Lower the heat, cover part-way let cook for 20 minutes.

16. Transfer to serving bowls and garnish with fresh parsley.

17. Serve and enjoy place over couscous.

Jeweled couscous recipe with pomegranate and lentils

This recipe combines mushrooms, lentil, nuts and raisins for a gorgeous dish the Mediterranean Sea way for a vegan.

Ingredients

- Salt
- ½ teaspoon of turmeric spice
- Olive oil
- 8 oz. mushrooms, cleaned and sliced
- 3 garlic cloves, chopped
- 1 teaspoon of sweet paprika
- 1 ⅔ cup of vegetable broth
- Water
- ½ teaspoon of ground green cardamom
- ½ teaspoon of ground coriander
- 1 cup of lentils
- 1 cup of gold raisins
- ½ cup of shelled chopped pistachios
- ½ teaspoon of ground cumin
- 2 cups of instant couscous
- 1 bunch of fresh mint stems removed, chopped

- ½ teaspoon of freshly ground black pepper
- 2 tablespoons of pomegranate molasses
- Juice of ½ lemon
- 1 bunch of fresh parsley, stems removed, chopped
- 1 small red onion, chopped
- 1 ½ teaspoon of ground cinnamon
- 6 scallions, tops trimmed, chopped
- Seeds of 1 large pomegranate
- 10 Medjool dates , pitted, chopped

Directions

1. Wash the lentils under running water. Drain.
2. Place the lentils in a saucepan and add 3 cups of water let boil, then reduce to simmer for 30 minutes.
3. Add a pinch of salt and remove from heat.
4. In a saucepan, bring the vegetable broth to a boil.
5. Stir in couscous together with the turmeric, pinch of salt, olive oil.
6. Cover and let sit 5 minutes to finish cooking.
7. In a large cast iron skillet, heat 2 tablespoons of olive oil.
8. Add the mushrooms let cook for 4 minutes on high, tossing occasionally.
9. Reduce heat to medium-high, and stir the onions and garlic and cook briefly.

10. In the same skillet, add in the cooked lentils and couscous.
11. Add salt together with the cinnamon, cardamom, paprika, coriander, and black pepper.
12. Mix the pomegranate molasses and lemon juice with 1 tablespoon of olive oil.
13. Add the liquid to the skillet with the couscous and lentil mixture. Toss to combine.
14. Let cook on medium, stirring regularly to warm through.
15. Remove from the heat, add the remaining ingredients.
16. Move the couscous to a serving platter.
17. Serve and enjoy.

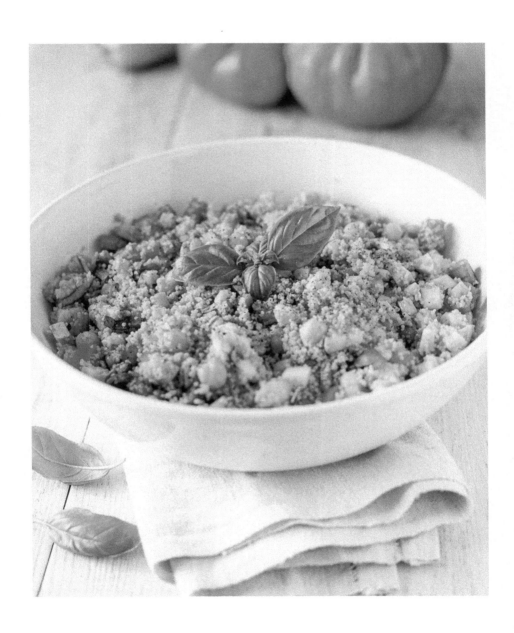

Lightning Source UK Ltd.
Milton Keynes UK
UKHW020842040621
384920UK00001B/64